Rise Above Breast Cancer

A Holistic Guide to Thriving Beyond Diagnosis

Jessica Luth

Copyright

Table of Content

Introduction

Getting Over Breast Cancer

When someone tells you, "You have breast cancer," everything stops. Your mind can be filled with a lot of different feelings, like fear, confusion, and anger. Having too much to handle is completely normal. The news of this illness changes my life, but it's also the start of a new journey. You're not alone on this trip.

Breast cancer is a hard road to travel, but you can get through it with strength, hope, and a healthy, whole-person attitude. This book will help you through every step by giving you information, support, and useful tips. Our goal is to help you rise above your diagnosis, not just live, but truly thrive.

Let's start by knowing that while breast cancer is a serious condition, many women have successfully fought it and come out stronger. Advances in medicine, along with a deeper knowledge of holistic health, provide us with powerful tools to combat this disease. This book combines conventional medical treatments with functional medicine approaches, giving you a complete guide to healing and wellness.

A holistic approach to breast cancer means looking at your health as a whole, not just focused on the disease itself. It's about supporting your body, mind, and spirit. This method emphasizes the value of lifestyle changes, mental and emotional support, and complementary therapies alongside traditional medical treatments.

1. Mindset and Mental Health

Your mindset plays a key role in your journey. Staying positive, maintaining hope, and managing stress are all important. Techniques such as mindfulness, meditation, and positive statements can help keep your mind strong and focused. Support groups and counseling can also provide emotional stability and a feeling of community.

2. Nutrition and Diet

What you eat greatly impacts your health. A balanced, nutrient-rich food can support your body's healing processes. We'll guide you through what to eat, when to eat, and how to make meals that are both delicious and beneficial. Foods rich in antioxidants, vitamins, and minerals can boost your defense system and energy levels.

3. Exercise and Physical Activity

Staying active is important. Exercise can help reduce fatigue, improve mood, and enhance general well-being. It doesn't have to be intense—gentle activities like walking, yoga, or swimming can be incredibly helpful. The key is to find something you enjoy and make it a regular part of your practice.

4. Sleep and Rest

Restorative sleep is a cornerstone of good health. Quality sleep helps your body heal, strengthens your immune system, and improves mental clarity. We'll explore tips and techniques to ensure you get the restful sleep your body needs, from building a relaxing bedtime routine to natural remedies that aid sleep.

5. Connection and Purpose

Humans are social creatures, and connections with others can provide immense mental support. Whether it's family, friends, or support groups, surrounding yourself with a strong support network is important. Additionally, finding a sense of purpose—whether through hobbies, volunteering, or personal projects—can give you drive and joy.

6. Integrative Therapies and Treatments

Beyond standard treatments like surgery, chemotherapy, and radiation, there are many complementary therapies that can support your healing. These include acupuncture, massage treatment, and herbal supplements. Each has its own benefits and can be integrated into your general treatment plan.

7. Personalized Medicine

Every person is unique, and so is every case of breast cancer. Personalized medicine tailors treatments to your specific genetic makeup and the traits of your cancer. This approach can improve the effectiveness of treatments and lessen side effects.

8. Education and Advocacy

Knowledge is power. Understanding your diagnosis, treatment choices, and the science behind breast cancer can empower you to make informed decisions about your health. Advocacy—speaking up for your wants and rights—ensures you receive the best possible care.

Every person's experience with breast cancer is different. Your journey is truly yours, influenced by your body, your emotions, your support system, and your beliefs. This book recognizes that individuality. It's not about having a one-size-fits-all plan; it's about finding what works best for you.

We'll teach you to listen to your body and trust your instincts. Your body has an amazing capacity for healing, and by supporting it with the right care and nourishment, you can improve this natural process.

Remember, you're not alone. There are countless women who have walked this path before you and countless others who are walking it now. Sharing your experiences, learning from others, and finding strength in community are important aspects of this journey. Support groups, both in-person and online, can provide a safe place to share, learn, and connect.

As you turn the pages of this book, take it one step at a time. You don't have to absorb everything at once. Let the information sink in gradually. Reflect on what connects with you and take action where you feel ready. Small, consistent steps can lead to major changes.

Rising above breast cancer is about taking a holistic approach to your health and well-being. It's about nurturing your body, mind, and spirit, and finding strength in every part of your life. This journey is challenging, but with the right help and mindset, it's one you can navigate successfully. Here's to your strength, your resilience, and your holistic path to health.

Chapter 1: What is Breast Cancer?

Breast cancer starts when cells in the breast begin to grow rapidly. These cells usually form a growth that can often be seen on an x-ray or felt as a lump. The tumor is called malignant (cancer) if the cells can invade surrounding tissues or spread to other parts of the body. While breast cancer is mainly a disease affecting women, men can develop it too, though it's much rarer.

The human breast is made up of glands, ducts, and connective parts. The glands, known as lobules, are where milk is made, and the ducts are the pathways that carry the milk to the nipple. Breast cancer usually originates in the cells lining these lobules or ducts.

The exact cause of breast cancer is not fully known, but several factors can increase the risk. These include genetic mutations (such as BRCA1 and BRCA2), hormonal changes, lifestyle factors (like diet and exercise), and environmental effects. It's important to remember that having risk factors does not mean you will definitely develop breast cancer, just as some people with breast cancer may not have any known risk factors.

Types and Stages of Breast Cancer

Breast cancer is not a single disease but a group of conditions with different traits. Understanding the types and stages of breast cancer can help you grasp the nature of the disease and the treatment choices available.

Types of Breast Cancer:

1. Ductal Carcinoma In Situ (DCIS): This is a non-invasive cancer where abnormal cells are found in the lining of a breast duct but haven't spread outside the duct. It's called the earliest form of breast cancer and is highly treatable.

2. Invasive Ductal Carcinoma (IDC): This is the most common type of breast cancer. It starts in the milk tubes and then invades nearby tissue in the breast. It can also spread to other parts of the body.

3. Invasive Lobular Carcinoma (ILC): This cancer starts in the lobules (milk-producing glands) and can spread to surrounding tissues. It's the second most common type of invasive breast cancer.

4. Triple-Negative Breast Cancer: This type misses three common receptors known to fuel most breast cancer growth—estrogen, progesterone, and the HER-2/neu gene. It's more difficult to treat because hormonal therapy and drugs that target HER-2 are ineffective.

5. HER2-Positive Breast Cancer: This cancer has a high amount of HER2 protein, which promotes the growth of cancer cells. Treatments that target the HER2 protein are helpful against this type.

6. Inflammatory Breast Cancer: A rare but aggressive form of breast cancer, it makes the breast look red and swollen because the cancer cells block lymph vessels in the skin.

7. Paget's Disease of the Nipple: This rare form starts in the tubes of the nipple but spreads to the nipple surface and the areola.

Stages of Breast Cancer:

Staging describes the extent of cancer within the body and is important in determining the prognosis and treatment plan. Here's a quick overview of the stages:

1. Stage 0: Known as carcinoma in situ, where cancer cells are limited to the ducts (DCIS) or lobules and have not spread.

2. Stage I: Early-stage invasive cancer where the tumor is up to 2 centimeters and has not spread to lymph nodes, or only has tiny amounts of cancer cells in lymph nodes.

3. Stage II: The growth is larger (2-5 centimeters) and/or has spread to a few nearby lymph nodes.

4. Stage III: More extensive spread to lymph nodes and probably chest wall or skin, but not to distant organs.

5. Stage IV: Cancer has spread to other parts of the body, such as bones, liver, lungs, or

brain. This is also known as spread breast cancer.

Each stage guides the treatment approach and helps predict outcomes.

Common Symptoms and Early Detection

Early detection of breast cancer significantly improves the chances of successful treatment. Being aware of the typical symptoms and regularly performing self-exams can help catch the disease in its early stages.

Common Symptoms of Breast Cancer:

1. Lump in the Breast or Underarm: The most common sign is a new lump or mass. While many lumps are benign, any new or unusual mass should be examined by a doctor.

2. Changes in Breast Shape or Size: Any obvious changes in the shape or size of the breast should be checked out.

3. Skin Changes: This can include dimpling, puckering, or swelling. The skin may also look pitted like an orange peel.

4. Nipple Changes: This includes changes in look, such as inversion (turning inward), or

discharge that isn't breast milk, especially if it's bloody.

5. Breast Pain: While most breast cancers don't cause pain, persistent pain or discomfort should be examined.

6. Swelling: Swelling of all or part of a breast, even if no lump is felt, can be a sign of breast cancer.

Early Detection:

1. Self-Exams: Regular self-examinations help you become familiar with your breasts' normal look and feel, so you can notice any changes early. It's usually recommended to do this once a month.

2. Clinical Breast Exams: During regular check-ups, your doctor can perform a clinical breast exam to check for lumps or other changes.

3. Mammograms: These are X-ray images of the breast used to identify early signs of cancer, often before a lump can be felt. Women over the age of 40 are usually advised to get a mammogram annually, but this can vary based on personal and family medical history.

4. Ultrasound and MRI: These imaging tests can be used alongside mammograms for a more thorough view, especially in women with dense breast tissue or higher risk factors.

5. Genetic Testing: For those with a family history of breast cancer, genetic testing for mutations like BRCA1 and BRCA2 can provide information about their risk and guide preventive steps.

By knowing what breast cancer is, recognizing the types and stages, and being vigilant about early detection, you can take proactive steps in managing your health. Remember, early discovery saves lives, so regular check-ups and being aware of your body are crucial. Together, we can rise above breast cancer, armed with knowledge, support, and a holistic approach to health.

Chapter 2: How Can Breast Cancer Be Treated?

When it comes to treating breast cancer, standard methods have been the cornerstone for many years. These methods include surgery, radiation, and chemotherapy. Each plays a unique role in managing the disease, and often, a mix of these treatments is used.

Surgery

Surgery is often the first line of treatment for breast cancer. The goal is to remove as much of the cancer as possible. There are different types of breast cancer surgeries, based on the extent and location of the cancer:

1.   Lumpectomy: Also   known   as breast-conserving surgery, a lumpectomy includes removing the cancerous tumor and a small margin of surrounding healthy tissue. This option is usually used for smaller tumors and aims to preserve as much of the breast as possible.

2. Mastectomy: In this operation, the entire breast is removed. There are different types of mastectomies, such as simple mastectomy (removal of the whole breast but not the lymph nodes under the arm), and modified radical mastectomy (removal of the whole breast and most of the lymph nodes under the arm).

3. Sentinel Lymph Node Biopsy: This surgery finds and removes the first few lymph nodes into which a tumor drains (sentinel nodes) to check for cancer spread. If these nodes are cancer-free, it's unlikely the cancer has spread to other lymph nodes.

4. Axillary Lymph Node Dissection: If cancer is found in the sentinel nodes, further surgery to remove extra lymph nodes (axillary dissection) might be necessary.

Radiation Therapy

Radiation therapy uses high-energy waves to target and kill cancer cells. It's often used after surgery to eliminate any leftover cancer cells in the breast, chest wall, or axilla (underarm area). The two main types of radiation treatment are:

1. External Beam Radiation: The most common form of radiation treatment, where a machine directs radiation beams to the cancer site from outside the body. Treatments are generally given five days a week over several weeks.

2. Internal Radiation (Brachytherapy): This includes placing radioactive material inside the body, near the cancer cells. It's less common and generally considered for specific cases.

Chemotherapy

Chemotherapy uses strong drugs to kill cancer cells or stop them from growing and dividing. It can be administered before surgery (neoadjuvant chemotherapy) to shrink tumors, making them easier to remove, or after surgery (adjuvant chemotherapy) to kill any remaining cancer cells and lower the risk of recurrence. Chemotherapy can also be used for advanced-stage breast cancer to treat the disease and improve symptoms.

Chemotherapy drugs are usually given intravenously (IV), but some can be taken orally. Treatment is usually given in cycles, with rest times in between to allow the body to recover.

Integrative Medicine: Combining Conventional and Holistic Approaches

Integrative medicine blends conventional cancer treatments with complementary therapies to address the whole person—body, mind, and spirit. This method can enhance the effectiveness of traditional treatments, reduce side effects, and improve general well-being.

Nutrition and Diet

A well-balanced diet plays a key role in supporting your body during cancer treatment. Eating a range of nutrient-rich foods can help boost your immune system, maintain strength, and promote healing. Here are some nutritional guidelines:

1. Eat Plenty of Fruits and Vegetables: These are rich in antioxidants, vitamins, and minerals that can help fight cancer and support general health.

2. Choose Whole Grains: Foods like brown rice, quinoa, and whole wheat bread provide important nutrients and fiber.

3. Include Lean Proteins: Sources like chicken, fish, beans, and nuts are important for muscle repair and defensive function.

4. Stay Hydrated: Drink plenty of water and avoid sugary drinks. Herbal teas can also be helpful.

Exercise and Physical Activity

Regular physical exercise can improve your physical and emotional health during and after cancer treatment. Exercise helps reduce fatigue, improve mood, and maintain a healthy weight. Activities such as walking, yoga, and swimming are excellent choices. Always consult your doctor before starting any new exercise routine.

Mind-Body Practices

Mind-body therapies can help handle stress, anxiety, and depression, which are common among breast cancer patients. Practices like meditation, mindfulness, and deep breathing movements foster relaxation and mental clarity. Techniques such as guided imagery, where you visualize happy outcomes, can also be helpful.

Acupuncture and Massage Therapy

Acupuncture includes inserting thin needles into specific points on the body to relieve pain and reduce side effects like nausea and fatigue. Massage therapy can alleviate stress, improve circulation, and help control pain and muscle tension. Both therapies can be useful additions to your treatment plan.

Herbal Supplements and Vitamins

Certain herbs and vitamins can help your body's healing process. However, it's important to consult with your healthcare provider before starting any supplements, as some can interact with cancer treatments. Common vitamins include:

1. Omega-3 Fatty Acids: Found in fish oil, these can help reduce inflammation and improve general health.

2. Vitamin D: Supports bone health and immune function.

3. Turmeric (Curcumin): Has anti-inflammatory effects that may help fight cancer cells.

Emerging Therapies and Innovations

Research and innovation in breast cancer treatment are continuing, leading to new therapies and better outcomes. Here are some of the biggest advancements:

Targeted Therapy

Targeted treatments focus on specific molecules involved in cancer growth and spread. Unlike chemotherapy, which affects all quickly dividing cells, targeted therapies aim at cancer-specific pathways. Examples include:

1. HER2-Targeted Therapy: Drugs like trastuzumab (Herceptin) target the HER2 protein, which supports the growth of some breast cancers.

2. CDK4/6 Inhibitors: These drugs, such as palbociclib (Ibrance), inhibit proteins that cause cell division in hormone receptor-positive breast cancers.

Immunotherapy

Immunotherapy helps the immune system detect and attack cancer cells. While still relatively new in breast cancer treatment, it has shown promise, especially in triple-negative breast cancer. Drugs like pembrolizumab (Keytruda) have been cleared for use in certain cases.

PARP Inhibitors

PARP inhibitors, such as olaparib (Lynparza), stop a protein used by cells to repair damage to their DNA. This makes it harder for cancer cells, especially those with BRCA mutations, to repair themselves, leading to cell death.

Liquid Biopsies

Liquid biopsies involve analyzing a blood sample to identify cancer DNA. This non-invasive method can help monitor cancer progression, spot recurrence early, and guide treatment choices.

Personalized Medicine

Advances in genomics and molecular biology have paved the way for personalized treatment. By analyzing a patient's genetic makeup and the specific characteristics of their cancer, treatments can be tailored to achieve the best results. This method helps identify which patients will benefit most from certain therapies, minimizing unnecessary side effects.

Treating breast cancer is a multifaceted process that needs a mix of conventional treatments, integrative approaches, and emerging therapies. Each patient's journey is unique, and a personalized treatment plan can provide the best chance for a successful result.

Chapter 3: How, When, and What to Eat

Nutritional Guidelines for Breast Cancer Patients

Nutrition plays a key role in supporting your body during and after breast cancer treatment. Eating a healthy, balanced diet can help manage treatment side effects, boost your immune system, and improve your general well-being. Here are some important nutritional guidelines for breast cancer patients:

1. Focus on Whole Foods: Aim to eat whole, raw foods as much as possible. These include fresh fruits and veggies, whole

grains, lean proteins, and healthy fats. Whole foods are rich in important nutrients that help your body heal and stay strong.

2. Increase Fruit and Vegetable Intake: Fruits and veggies are packed with vitamins, minerals, and antioxidants that can help protect your cells from damage. Aim for a range of colors and types to get a broad spectrum of nutrients.

3. Choose Lean Proteins: Protein is important for repairing tissues and maintaining muscle mass, especially during cancer treatment. Good sources of lean protein include chicken, turkey, fish, beans, lentils, and tofu.

4. Opt for Healthy Fats: Healthy fats, such as those found in avocados, nuts, seeds, and olive oil, can help lower inflammation and provide long-lasting energy. Avoid trans fats and reduce saturated fats.

5. Stay Hydrated: Drinking plenty of water is crucial for general health and can help alleviate some treatment side effects like dry mouth and fatigue. Aim for at least 8-10 glasses of water a day.

6. Limit Sugar and Processed Foods: High sugar intake and processed foods can lead to weight gain and other health problems. Try to minimize your intake of sweets, sugary drinks, and highly processed snacks.

7. Monitor Portion Sizes: Eating the right portion sizes helps maintain a healthy weight, which is important for general health and can impact cancer prognosis. Listen to your body's food cues and avoid overeating.

Superfoods and Their Benefits

Certain foods are particularly useful for their high nutrient content and health-promoting properties. These superfoods can play an important role in a breast cancer patient's diet:

1. Berries: Blueberries, strawberries, and raspberries are rich in antioxidants, which can help protect your cells from damage.

They also contain vitamins and fiber, supporting general health.

2. Leafy Greens: Spinach, kale, and Swiss chard are packed with vitamins A, C, and K, as well as folate and fiber. These nutrients support immune function and general health.

3. Cruciferous Vegetables: Broccoli, cauliflower, and Brussels sprouts contain compounds like sulforaphane, which have been shown to have cancer-fighting qualities.

4. Nuts and Seeds: Almonds, walnuts, chia seeds, and flaxseeds provide healthy fats, protein, and fiber. They also contain antioxidants and other compounds that can help lower inflammation.

5. Fish: Fatty fish like salmon, mackerel, and sardines are rich in omega-3 fatty acids, which can help lower inflammation and support heart health.

6. Turmeric: This spice contains curcumin, which has anti-inflammatory and antioxidant qualities. Adding turmeric to your meals can improve flavor and provide health benefits.

7. Green Tea: Rich in antioxidants called catechins, green tea has been shown to have cancer-fighting qualities. Drinking green tea regularly can help overall health.

8. Garlic: Garlic contains compounds like allicin, which have been shown to have cancer-fighting qualities. It also helps immune function and cardiovascular health.

Creating a Balanced and Healing Meal Plan

Developing a meal plan that includes these nutritional guidelines and superfoods can help you stay on track and ensure you're getting the nutrients you need. Here are some tips for making a balanced and healing meal plan:

1. Plan Ahead: Take time each week to plan your meals and snacks. This can help you make healthier choices and escape the temptation of processed or fast foods.

2. Balance Your Plate: Aim to fill half your plate with veggies and fruits, a quarter with lean protein, and a quarter with whole

grains. This balance ensures you're getting a range of nutrients.

3. Include a Variety of Foods: Eating a wide range of foods helps you get a broad variety of nutrients. Try to add different fruits, vegetables, proteins, and grains into your meals.

4. Snack Smart: Choose healthy snacks like nuts, seeds, yogurt, or veggies to keep your energy levels stable throughout the day. Avoid sugary or processed snacks.

5. Experiment with Recipes: Look for healthy recipes that combine superfoods and other nutritious products. Trying new recipes can keep your meals interesting and pleasant.

6. Listen to Your Body: Pay attention to how different things make you feel. Some foods may cause pain or other side effects, especially during treatment. Adjust your food based on your body's responses.

Here's a sample day of meals:

Breakfast:

- Smoothie with spinach,
- blueberries,
- a banana, chia seeds,
- and almond milk.

Mid-Morning Snack:

- Greek yogurt with a handful of walnuts
- and a drop of honey.

Lunch:

- Quinoa salad with mixed greens,
- cherry tomatoes, cucumbers, beans,
- and a lemon-tahini dressing.

Afternoon Snack:

Apple slices with almond butter.

Dinner:

Baked salmon with a side of roasted Brussels sprouts and sweet potatoes.

Evening Snack: Green tea and a piece of dark chocolate.

Timing Your Meals for Optimal Health

When you eat can be just as important as what you eat. Proper meal timing can help keep your energy levels, support digestion, and improve overall health. Here are some tips for timing your meals:

1. Eat Regularly: Try to eat three big meals and two to three small snacks throughout the day. Eating regularly helps keep your blood sugar levels stable and stops overeating.

2. Don't Skip Breakfast: Breakfast kickstarts your metabolism and gives energy for the day ahead. Include protein, whole grains, and fruits or veggies in your morning meal.

3. Fuel Before and After Workouts: If you're training, have a small snack that includes carbohydrates and protein about 30 minutes before your workout. After exercising, eat a meal or snack with protein to help your muscles heal.

4. Avoid Late-Night Eating: Eating too close to bedtime can upset your sleep and digestion. Try to finish your last meal at least two to three hours before going to bed.

5. Stay Hydrated Throughout the Day: Drinking water regularly throughout the day can help keep hydration and support digestion. Carry a water bottle with you to remember yourself to drink.

6. Listen to Your Hunger Cues: Pay attention to your body's signs of hunger and fullness. Eat when you're hungry, and stop when you're full. This can help avoid overeating and support healthy digestion.

By following these nutritional guidelines, incorporating superfoods, making balanced meal plans, and timing your meals properly, you can support your body's healing process during and after breast cancer treatment. Remember, every person's journey is unique, so it's important to listen to your body and change your diet as needed. With a mindful approach to eating, you can nourish your body, boost your energy levels, and improve your general well-being.

Chapter 4: The Secret to Nourishing Sleep

Sleep is a basic pillar of health and well-being, especially when you're dealing with a condition like breast cancer. Quality sleep is important for your body to repair and rejuvenate. During sleep, your body works hard to heal tissues, build bone and muscle, and improve your immune system. For breast cancer patients, sleep is particularly important for several reasons:

1. Boosts Immune Function: Sleep helps regulate your immune system, which is important in fighting cancer and reducing the risk of infections.

2. Reduces Inflammation: Poor sleep can increase inflammation in the body, which may add to cancer progression. Adequate sleep helps keep inflammation in check.

3. Supports Mental Health: Battling cancer can be physically taxing. Good sleep helps regulate mood, reduce stress, and improve mental clarity, making it easier to cope with the emotional difficulties.

4. Enhances Treatment Efficacy: Sleep allows your body to react better to cancer treatments like chemotherapy and radiation, possibly enhancing their effectiveness.

5. Aids Recovery: Post-surgery and treatment, your body needs sleep to repair tissues and heal more quickly.

Creating a Restful Sleep Environment

Creating a sleep-friendly environment can make a major difference in the quality of your sleep. Here are some tips to help you set up a restful sleep space:

1. Comfortable Bedding: Invest in a good quality mattress and blankets that provide adequate support and comfort. Soft, airy sheets and blankets can also improve your sleep quality.

2. Darkness: Ensure your bedroom is as dark as possible. Use blackout curtains or an eye mask to block out light, which can interfere with your sleep routine.

3. Quiet: Minimize noise disturbances by using earplugs or a white noise machine. A quiet setting helps your brain relax and stay in a deep sleep.

4. Cool Temperature: Keep your bedroom cool, ideally between 60-67 degrees Fahrenheit (15-19 degrees Celsius). A cool environment helps your body control its temperature, promoting better sleep.

5. Declutter: A clean, uncluttered room can have a calming effect. Keep your bedroom tidy and free of distractions like work tools or clutter.

6. Limit Electronics: Avoid using tech devices like phones, tablets, and TVs in the

bedroom. The blue light released from screens can interfere with your body's production of melatonin, the hormone that regulates sleep.

7. Relaxing smells: Consider using calming smells like lavender or chamomile. Essential oils or scented candles can create a soothing environment conducive to sleep.

Natural Remedies for Better Sleep

Sometimes, despite making a restful environment, you may still find it challenging to sleep well. Natural remedies can be a gentle way to improve sleep quality without counting on medication:

1. Herbal Teas: Teas made from herbs like chamomile, valerian root, and passionflower have natural sedative effects that can help you relax and fall asleep more easily.

2. Magnesium Supplements: Magnesium is a mineral that helps regulate sleep by calming the nervous system. Foods rich in magnesium (such as leafy veggies, nuts, and seeds) or a magnesium supplement can help improve sleep quality.

3. Melatonin Supplements: Melatonin is a hormone that affects sleep-wake cycles. A melatonin supplement can be particularly helpful if you're experiencing disruptions in your sleep routine. However, ask your doctor before starting any new supplement.

4. Aromatherapy: Essential oils like lavender, bergamot, and sandalwood can promote calm and improve sleep. Use a diffuser, or add a few drops to a warm bath before bed.

5. Meditation and Deep Breathing:
Practicing mindfulness meditation or deep breathing exercises can help calm your mind and prepare your body for sleep. These methods reduce stress and promote relaxation, making it easier to fall asleep and stay asleep.

6. Warm Bath: Taking a warm bath an hour or two before bed can help relax your muscles and lower your body temperature, signaling to your body that it's time to sleep.

7. Limit Caffeine and Alcohol: Both caffeine and alcohol can disrupt sleep habits. Try to avoid caffeine in the afternoon and evening, and limit alcohol intake, as it can affect the quality of your sleep.

Managing Sleep Disruptions and Insomnia

Sleep disruptions and insomnia are typical issues, especially for those undergoing cancer treatment. Here are some strategies to help handle these challenges:

1. Consistent Sleep Schedule: Go to bed and wake up at the same time every day, even on

weekends. A regular sleep plan helps regulate your internal clock.

2. Wind-Down habit: Establish a relaxing pre-sleep habit to signal to your body that it's time to unwind. This could include reading a book, taking a warm bath, or performing gentle yoga.

3. Limit Naps: While it's important to listen to your body, try to limit naps to 20-30 minutes and avoid napping late in the day, as it can interfere with nighttime sleep.

4. Stay Active: Regular physical exercise can help you fall asleep faster and enjoy deeper sleep. Aim for at least 30 minutes of

moderate exercise most days, but avoid vigorous action close to bedtime.

5. Manage Stress: Techniques like journaling, talking to a friend, or getting support from a therapist can help you manage stress and anxiety, which often contribute to sleep problems.

6. Mindfulness and Relaxation Techniques: Practices like progressive muscle relaxation, guided images, and mindfulness meditation can help you relax and ease into sleep.

7. Limit Fluids Before Bed: To lower the need for nighttime bathroom trips, try to limit fluid intake in the hours leading up to bedtime.

8. Seek Professional Help: If you've tried these techniques and are still struggling with sleep, it may be time to seek help from a healthcare provider. They can check for underlying conditions and provide additional treatment options, such as cognitive-behavioral therapy for insomnia (CBT-I).

Good sleep supports your physical, emotional, and mental health, helping you feel more energized and better able to face the challenges of breast cancer treatment and recovery.

Chapter 5: The Power of Connection and Purpose

Going through breast cancer treatment can be an incredibly isolating experience, but it doesn't have to be. Building a supportive community around you is important for emotional well-being and can significantly impact your healing journey. Here's how to develop a network of support:

Reach Out to Family and Friends

Your family and friends can be your first line of support. They love you and want to help, but sometimes they might not know how. Don't hesitate to voice your needs and let them know how they can assist you, whether it's through practical help, like cooking meals and running errands, or emotional support, like listening to you talk about your feelings and fears.

Join Support Groups

Connecting with others who are going through similar situations can be incredibly comforting. Support groups, both in-person and online, offer a space to share your story, gain insights from others, and receive support from those who truly understand what you're going through. Look for local cancer support groups, or explore internet forums and social media groups dedicated to breast cancer survivors.

Seek Professional Support

Sometimes, professional help is important. Psychologists, counselors, and social workers specializing in cancer care can provide invaluable emotional support and coping techniques. They can help you navigate the complex feelings that come with a cancer diagnosis and treatment, such as fear, anger, sadness, and anxiety.

Connect with Fellow Patients

In your treatment center, you'll likely meet other patients going through similar paths. Don't be afraid to strike up talks in the waiting room or during chemotherapy sessions. These connections can lead to lasting friendships and mutual support that extend beyond the treatment time.

Leverage Technology

In today's digital age, technology can be a powerful tool for building and keeping connections. Use video calls to stay in touch with distant loved ones, join virtual support groups, and connect with online communities through social media platforms and dedicated cancer support websites.

Participate in Community Activities

Engaging in community activities, like volunteering or joining local clubs, can provide a feeling of normalcy and help you stay connected with the world outside of your illness. Activities that match with your interests can also offer a mental break from the stresses of treatment.

Finding Meaning and Purpose in Your Journey

Breast cancer can be a life-altering experience, but it can also be a chance to find new meaning and purpose. Here are ways to discover greater significance in your journey:

Reflect on Your Life Priorities

A cancer diagnosis often prompts a reevaluation of life's goals. Take time to think on what truly matters to you. This might involve spending more time with loved ones, following passions that you've neglected, or letting go of things that no longer serve you.

Set Meaningful Goals

Setting goals can give you a sense of direction and purpose. These goals don't have to be grand or ambitious; they can be small, daily objectives that give you a sense of success. Whether it's finishing a book, learning a new sport, or simply getting through a tough day, each goal achieved is a step forward.

Find Joy in Helping Others

Helping others can be incredibly rewarding and can shift your attention away from your own struggles. Consider volunteering for causes you care about, mentoring someone who's newly diagnosed, or simply giving a listening ear to others in need. Acts of kindness and service can provide a profound sense of purpose and satisfaction.

Pursue Creative Outlets

Engaging in creative activities, like drawing, writing, music, or crafting, can be therapeutic. These activities allow you to express your feelings, process your experiences, and find joy in the act of creation. Creative activities can also serve as a form of escapism, providing a mental break from the stresses of cancer.

Practice Gratitude

Focusing on the positive aspects of your life, no matter how small, can greatly impact your outlook. Keeping a gratitude journal, where you jot down things you're thankful for each day, can help shift your mindset from one of scarcity to one of wealth. Gratitude practices can promote resilience and a deeper appreciation for life's simple pleasures.

Engage in Mindfulness and Meditation

Mindfulness and meditation techniques can help you stay present and find peace amid the chaos. These techniques encourage you to focus on the here and now, reducing stress and anxiety. Meditation can also help you connect with your inner self, giving clarity and insight into your life's purpose.

Embrace Spirituality

For many, faith is a source of strength and comfort. Whether it's through religious practices, meditation, nature walks, or personal reflection, connecting with your spiritual beliefs can provide a sense of meaning and help you deal with the challenges of cancer.

Celebrate Milestones

Acknowledging and celebrating your success, no matter how small, is important. Each treatment finished, each positive scan, and each personal victory is a milestone worth celebrating. These celebrations reinforce your resilience and provide motivation to keep going forward.

Connect with Nature

Spending time in nature can be incredibly healing. Whether it's a walk in the park, gardening, or simply sitting outside and soaking up the sun, nature has a way of grounding us and telling us of life's beauty. It can provide a sense of peace and renewal that is important during challenging times.

Document Your Journey

Writing about your events can be a powerful tool for finding meaning. Whether it's through journaling, blogging, or creating a memoir, documenting your trip allows you to process your thoughts and feelings. It can also serve as a source of inspiration and comfort to others who read your story.

The power of connection and purpose cannot be overstated, especially when facing a challenging path like breast cancer. Building a supportive community and finding meaning in your experiences are important components of emotional and mental well-being.

Chapter 5: Supplements, Treatments

When fighting breast cancer, many patients look for ways to complement their conventional treatments. Supplements can play a major role in supporting your body during this time.

However, it's crucial to speak with your healthcare provider before adding any supplements to your regimen, as they can interact with medications and treatments. Here are some nutrients that are often recommended for breast cancer patients:

Vitamin D

Vitamin D is important for bone health and immune function. Research shows that it may also play a role in reducing the risk of breast cancer recurrence. Many people have low levels of vitamin D, especially during the winter months, so supplementation can be helpful. Aim for a blood test to determine your levels and suitable dosage.

Omega-3 Fatty Acids

Found in fish oil and flaxseed oil, omega-3 fatty acids have anti-inflammatory properties that can support general health. They may help reduce inflammation and improve heart health, which is especially important if you're undergoing treatments that can strain your cardiovascular system.

Curcumin

Curcumin, the active ingredient in turmeric, has strong anti-inflammatory and antioxidant properties. Some studies suggest that it can inhibit the growth of cancer cells and improve the effectiveness of chemotherapy. Consider adding turmeric to your diet or taking a curcumin supplement.

Probiotics

Chemotherapy and radiation can disrupt your gut flora, leading to digestive problems. Probiotics can help repair healthy bacteria in your gut, improving digestion and boosting your immune system. Look for a high-quality probiotic supplement with a range of strains.

Green Tea Extract

Green tea is rich in polyphenols, especially epigallocatechin gallate (EGCG), which has been shown to have anti-cancer properties. Drinking green tea or taking a green tea extract pill can provide these benefits. However, be careful with the dosage, as high amounts can interfere with certain medications.

Vitamin C

Vitamin C is a powerful antioxidant that can help your immune system. Some studies show high-dose vitamin C may enhance the effects of certain cancer treatments. It's available in various forms, including oral supplements and intravenous infusions, but the latter should only be given under medical supervision.

Milk Thistle

Milk thistle is widely used to support liver health. Since your liver processes many of the toxins from chemotherapy, keeping it healthy is important. Milk thistle's active ingredient, silymarin, has antioxidant effects that can help protect your liver from damage.

Mushroom Extracts

Certain mushrooms, such as reishi, shiitake, and maitake, contain substances that can boost your immune system. These mushrooms are available as nutrients and can support your body's natural defenses during treatment.

Coenzyme Q10 (CoQ10)

CoQ10 is an antioxidant that helps make energy in your cells. Chemotherapy can decrease your body's natural CoQ10 levels, so supplementation can help reduce fatigue and support heart health.

Exploring Alternative Therapies

While conventional treatments like surgery, chemotherapy, and radiation are important in treating breast cancer, many patients seek alternative therapies to complement their treatment plan. These therapies can help manage symptoms, lessen side effects, and improve quality of life. Here are some alternative treatments worth exploring:

Acupuncture

Acupuncture, a traditional Chinese medicine practice, includes inserting thin needles into specific points on the body. It can help alleviate pain, reduce nausea, and improve general well-being. Many cancer centers now offer acupuncture as part of their supportive care services.

Massage Therapy

Massage therapy can provide relief from muscle tension, improve circulation, and lower stress. It's important to seek a massage therapist who has experience working with cancer patients to ensure the methods used are safe and appropriate.

Yoga

Yoga blends physical postures, breathing exercises, and meditation. It can help improve flexibility, reduce stress, and boost emotional well-being. Gentle yoga classes designed for cancer patients can be particularly helpful.

Mind-Body Techniques

Practices like meditation, mindfulness, and guided imagery can help you handle stress and improve mental clarity. These techniques encourage relaxation and can reduce anxiety, improve sleep, and enhance your general sense of peace.

Herbal Medicine

Herbal medicine includes using plants and plant extracts to support health. While some herbs have shown promise in cancer care, it's important to consult with a knowledgeable practitioner. Some herbs can interact with conventional treatments or have side effects.

Naturopathy

Naturopathic medicine focuses on natural treatments and the body's power to heal itself. Naturopaths may suggest dietary changes, supplements, herbal remedies, and lifestyle modifications. Working with a naturopath skilled in oncology can provide personalized support.

Reiki

Reiki is a form of energy medicine that aims to balance the body's energy fields. A Reiki practitioner gently puts their hands on or near your body to promote relaxation and healing. While scientific proof is limited, many people find Reiki to be a comforting and stress-reducing practice.

Aromatherapy

Aromatherapy uses essential oils extracted from plants to support physical and emotional well-being. Oils like lavender, peppermint, and chamomile can be used in diffusers, applied to the skin (with a carrier oil), or added to baths. Aromatherapy can help reduce anxiety, improve mood, and increase relaxation.

Dietary Changes

Nutrition plays a key role in supporting your body during cancer treatment. Working with a nutritionist or dietitian who specializes in oncology can help you build a diet that meets your specific needs. Incorporating nutrient-dense foods, reducing sugar and processed foods, and staying hydrated are basic dietary principles.

Art Therapy

Engaging in artistic activities like painting, drawing, or crafting can be therapeutic. Art therapy helps you to express emotions that might be difficult to articulate with words. It can provide a feeling of accomplishment and serve as a mental escape from the rigors of treatment.

Homeopathy

Homeopathy is a method of natural medicine that uses highly diluted substances to stimulate the body's healing processes. While controversial and not widely accepted in mainstream medicine, some patients claim benefits from homeopathic treatments. It's important to consult a qualified homeopath.

Combining Conventional and Alternative Approaches

Integrating alternative therapies with standard care can provide a more holistic approach to managing breast cancer. Here's how to successfully combine these methods:

1. Communicate with Your Healthcare Team: Always tell your oncologist and other healthcare providers about any supplements or alternative therapies you're considering. This ensures they can advise on possible interactions and monitor your overall treatment plan.

2. Find Qualified Practitioners: Look for practitioners skilled in working with cancer patients. They can tailor treatments to your unique needs and ensure safety and efficacy.

3. Focus on Evidence-Based Practices: While studying alternative therapies, prioritize those with scientific support. Practices like acupuncture, massage treatment, and mindfulness have been

studied and shown to provide benefits for cancer patients.

4. Listen to Your Body: Pay attention to how your body responds to different treatments. What works for one person might not work for another, so it's important to find what feels best for you.

5. Maintain a Balanced Approach: Use alternative therapies to support, not replace, conventional treatments. An integrative method can enhance your overall well-being and improve your quality of life.

6. Stay Informed: Research and stay updated on new breakthroughs in both conventional and alternative cancer treatments.

Knowledge empowers you to make informed choices about your care.

Navigating breast cancer treatment can be overwhelming, but considering supplements, alternative therapies, and outside-of-the-box approaches can provide extra support and improve your quality of life. Always speak with your healthcare team before making any changes to your treatment plan to ensure safety and compatibility.

Case Studies: Success Stories and Lessons Learned

Real-life success stories can offer hope and important lessons for anyone navigating a breast cancer diagnosis. Here are a few inspiring cases of how personalized medicine has made a difference in the lives of breast cancer patients:

Case Study 1: Emily's Journey with BRCA Mutation

Emily, a 45-year-old mother of two, was diagnosed with breast cancer after a regular mammogram showed an abnormality. Genetic testing showed that Emily had a BRCA1 mutation, which significantly increased her risk for both breast and ovarian cancer. Armed with this information, her medical team created a personalized treatment plan that included a double mastectomy to reduce the risk of recurrence, followed by targeted therapy with a PARP inhibitor. This drug is particularly helpful for patients with BRCA mutations. Emily also underwent prophylactic oophorectomy to prevent ovarian cancer. Today, Emily is cancer-free and actively involved in raising knowledge about genetic testing and personalized treatment options.

Lessons Learned: The Importance of Genetic Testing: Emily's case shows the critical role of genetic testing in identifying high-risk patients and tailoring treatment plans accordingly.

- Proactive Measures: Preventative surgeries, while a difficult choice, can greatly reduce the risk of recurrence and improve long-term outcomes.

Case Study 2: John's Immunotherapy Success

John, a 52-year-old man, was identified with triple-negative breast cancer (TNBC), a particularly aggressive form of breast cancer that lacks hormone receptors and HER2 protein. Standard treatments for TNBC are limited, but genetic testing showed that John's tumor had a high level of PD-L1 protein, making him a good candidate for immunotherapy. John enrolled in a clinical study for an immunotherapy drug called pembrolizumab, which works by targeting the PD-L1 protein and boosting the immune system's ability to fight cancer. After several months of treatment, John's tumors shrank significantly, and he gained a partial remission. He continues to receive immunotherapy and is having a good quality of life.

Lessons Learned: The Potential of Immunotherapy: John's experience shows the potential of immunotherapy in treating hard-to-treat cancers like TNBC.

The Value of Clinical Trials: Participating in clinical studies can provide access to cutting-edge treatments that are not yet widely available.

Case Study 3: Lisa's Targeted Therapy Triumph

Lisa, a 38-year-old woman, was discovered with HER2-positive breast cancer, a type of cancer that grows quickly and is more likely to spread. HER2-positive cancers overexpress the HER2 protein, which supports the growth of cancer cells. Lisa's genetic test showed the overexpression of HER2, making her a candidate for targeted therapy with trastuzumab (Herceptin). This drug directly targets the HER2 protein, blocking its activity and slowing the growth of cancer cells. Lisa's treatment plan included trastuzumab in combination with chemotherapy. After finishing her treatment, Lisa's scans showed no evidence of disease, and she has been in remission for three years.

Lessons Learned: Effectiveness of Targeted Therapy: Lisa's case shows the power of targeted therapies in treating specific types of breast cancer.

- Combination Treatment: Combining targeted therapy with conventional treatments like chemotherapy can improve outcomes and lower the risk of recurrence.

Case Study 4: Rachel's Personalized Nutrition Plan

Rachel, a 50-year-old breast cancer survivor, was looking for ways to avoid recurrence and improve her overall health after completing her treatment. Her oncologist suggested a personalized nutrition plan based on genetic tests. The test showed that Rachel had specific genetic variants that affected her ability to process certain nutrients and increased her risk of inflammation.

With the help of a nutritionist, Rachel chose a diet rich in anti-inflammatory foods, such as fruits, vegetables, whole grains, and omega-3 fatty acids, while avoiding processed foods and sugars. She also started taking supplements suited to her genetic profile. Rachel reports feeling more energetic, keeping a healthy weight, and experiencing fewer digestive issues.

Lessons Learned: The Role of Nutrition: Personalized nutrition plans based on genetic insights can improve overall health and support cancer prevention.

- Holistic Approach: Addressing diet and lifestyle factors can play a major role in long-term cancer care.

Conclusion

A breast cancer diagnosis is life-changing, and even after treatment, the journey continues as you adjust to a new normal. This phase includes embracing changes, both physical and emotional, and finding ways to thrive beyond your diagnosis. Here's how you can handle this transition and live a fulfilling life after breast cancer:

Accepting Change

The first step in enjoying your new normal is accepting that change is inevitable. Whether it's physical changes like surgery scars or hair loss, or emotional changes such as anxiety about recurrence, acknowledging these shifts lets you to move forward.

Acceptance doesn't mean giving up; it means knowing that your life is different now and finding ways to adapt.

Finding Your New Routine

Creating a new daily routine can help create a sense of normalcy. This might include adopting healthy habits such as regular exercise, a balanced diet, and mindfulness practices. Setting up a consistent routine can provide structure and make it easier to manage any lingering side effects of treatment.

Focusing on Wellness

Wellness goes beyond physical health to include emotional, mental, and spiritual well-being. Engage in activities that bring you joy and lower stress, whether it's yoga, meditation, reading, or spending time with loved ones. Prioritizing self-care is important as you adjust to life after cancer.

Reconnecting with Yourself

Cancer can shift your outlook on life. Take time to think on what's important to you now. You might find new hobbies or rediscover old passions. Journaling, therapy, or support groups can help you explore these changes and set new goals for the future.

Your health journey doesn't end when treatment does. It's an ongoing process that needs attention and care. Here are some strategies to keep and enhance your health and well-being as you move forward:

Regular Health Check-ups

Continued medical follow-up is important. Regular check-ups with your oncologist and other healthcare providers help watch your recovery and catch any signs of recurrence early. Keep a schedule of your meetings and stay proactive about your health.

Healthy Eating

Nutrition plays a vital part in your long-term health. Focus on a diet high in fruits, vegetables, whole grains, and lean proteins. Avoid processed foods and extra sugars. A nutritionist or dietitian specializing in oncology can help you create a meal plan that supports your general health and reduces the risk of recurrence.

Exercise

Physical activity is good for both your body and mind. It can help you recover strength, improve mood, and reduce fatigue. Find things you enjoy, whether it's walking, swimming, dancing, or yoga. Aim for at least 150 minutes of moderate exercise each week, but listen to your body and change as needed.

Mental Health

Taking care of your mental health is just as important as your physical health. Therapy, counseling, or support groups can provide a safe place to express your feelings and cope with any emotional challenges. Practices like mindfulness and meditation can help reduce anxiety and improve general well-being.

Sleep

Quality sleep is important for healing and overall health. Establish a bedtime practice that promotes restful sleep. This might include winding down with a book, taking a warm bath, or practicing relaxation methods. Ensure your sleep surroundings is comfortable and free from distractions.

Stress Management

Stress can badly impact your health. Find effective ways to handle stress, such as deep breathing exercises, hobbies, or spending time in nature. Regularly practicing relaxation methods can help keep stress levels in check and improve your quality of life.

Thriving beyond a breast cancer diagnosis involves accepting your new normal, continuing your wellness journey, and seeking out resources for ongoing support and information. Remember, this is a race, not a sprint. Be patient with yourself, celebrate small wins, and prioritize your well-being.

About the Author

Jessica Luth's battle with breast cancer serves as an inspiration for tenacity, optimism, and the transforming potential of knowledge and community. As a survivor and an ardent advocate, Jessica has committed her life to encouraging people going through comparable struggles. Her background, together with her in-depth studies and dedication to holistic wellbeing, establish her as a reliable authority in the field of breast cancer support and awareness.

Jessica's story started with a regular mammography that revealed she had breast cancer. She was overcome with anxiety and uncertainty, much like many others. But Jessica discovered an inner strength that carried her over the initial shock. Dedicated to walking her journey with bravery and clarity, she engaged herself in learning every aspect of her diagnosis and available treatments.

Jessica took her medical care head-on, undergoing radiation, chemotherapy, and surgery. She relied on her loved ones, close friends, and a committed medical team throughout these trying times. Her recuperation was greatly aided by their steadfast support and her unwavering spirit.

Jessica became a champion for breast cancer education and awareness as a result of her experiences. She came to see that information is an effective weapon in the fight against cancer. She wants to use her advocacy to provide others access to the knowledge and tools that she didn't have when she started out.

Because of her commitment, Jessica has worked with numerous cancer support groups, taken part in awareness campaigns, and supported research projects. She has given speeches at various gatherings, using her experience and wisdom to uplift and inform the audience. Her mission is to demystify breast cancer and make essential information easily understood by anyone.

Beyond traditional medicine, Jessica investigated alternative methods of well-being. She supports a holistic approach to treatment that takes into account the mind, spirit, and body in addition to the physical body. Her book, in which she blends holistic methods with medical knowledge, reflects this belief.

Jessica has a strong foundation in both personal experience and in-depth study when it comes to integrative therapies, nutrition, and mindfulness. She promotes a balanced way of living that incorporates mental health services, regular exercise, a nutritious diet, and spiritual and mental well-being. Her holistic approach to life after cancer emphasizes thriving above only surviving.

Her journey from a cancer patient facing uncertainty to a strong survivor and advocate is a source of inspiration. She is aware of the anxiety, difficulties, and victories associated with receiving a breast cancer diagnosis. Her genuineness and sensitivity are contagious to everyone she speaks to or writes to. For anyone dealing with breast cancer, Jessica Luth's book serves as both a companion and a guide. She offers helpful counsel, genuine support, and reassurance that you are not alone. Her goal is to give others the courage and hope they need to overcome their diagnosis, accept their new normal, and carry on with their wellness path.

My goal in creating this book is to impart the wisdom and fortitude I've acquired from going through my personal breast cancer experience. Each action, difficulty, and accomplishment has molded me into the person I am today. I want to provide the tools and assistance that changed my life to others. By working together, we may bravely and resolutely traverse this journey and come out stronger than before." - Jessica Luth

I Have a Request

Dear Reader,

Thanks for your purchase,Hope you enjoyed reading. Could you please leave a positive feedback?

If you've found value in "Rise Above Breast Cancer: A holistic guide to thriving beyond diagnosis " we would love to hear from you! Your feedback not only helps us improve but also assists others in finding effective solutions for their knee pain. Please take a moment to leave a review and share your experience with the book.

Every piece of feedback is greatly appreciated and plays a crucial role in helping others on their journey to better health. Thank you for your support!